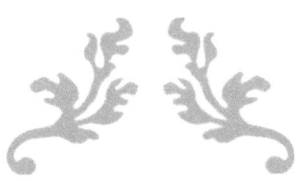

Living Life in the NICU

Insights and Perspectives

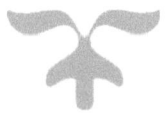

Patti Cleveland

ISBN 978-1-387-99128-0

This book is dedicated to all of those individuals who have dedicated their life and love to caring for and healing our children and supporting families who face challenges in their child's first days and years of life. It is a special calling and we thank you for answering the call.

Our Story

Pregnancy is considered to be a normal function of the circle of life, yet some of us have experiences that are far from normal. Pregnancy is a miraculous thing. It is so extraordinary to think just how many elements are at play and how they all have to occur just at the right time to bring a healthy baby into this world. Still, most mothers think that this type of event will never happen to them – myself included!

After two pregnancies that didn't survive the first 8 weeks, I was finally pregnant and progressing normally until my water broke during my 22nd week into the pregnancy. My husband rushed me to my local hospital when upon arrival, my contractions were 5 minutes apart! The doctors were able to get my contractions more in control, but if my baby would have any chance of survival we were going to have to be transported to a hospital where they had a Neonatal Intensive Care Unit. The nearest one was 50 miles away.

I had considered myself to be someone who was in control of their life, yet during pregnancy, it was abundantly clear what little control I actually had. I was simply providing the room and snacks! We still don't know exactly why Kayla came to us so early, but one thing was abundantly clear – she made the decision to be born and there was no holding her back!

Kayla allowed us 3 days of extra time from when my contractions started to her insistence on being born. When I was told that there was no more chance of holding off her birth, I knew I had one more task and then it was between Kayla and her Creator as to what her future would hold.

At 23 weeks gestation, there was not much data on what to expect and birth at that stage carried a myriad of possible outcomes. Once she was born, we became the stewards for her spirit. Having a baby so early is a situation that tends to paint a grim picture. Statistically, we started this process with a 10% chance of survival. With each day, we gained 3%. The possible outcomes for her included such things as major lung disease, blindness, brain bleeds leading to retardation, learning disabilities, and cerebral palsy –

just to name a few, a major few! She did have lung infections, surgery to close a valve in her heart at 9 days old, minor brain bleeds which caused concerns about her vision, and lung damage. This may sound daunting, but in the scheme of things, not unexpected nor abnormal. These children are very resilient and tend to have a fierce fighting spirit. They often outgrow the effects of these events. Through excellent care, prayer, and mamma's milk, after 142 days in the NICU, we took home a thriving baby.

We went home on oxygen and a monitor and I pumped breast milk for nine full months after we came home. We had some medications to administer at home, but with the education I received while in the NICU, I felt confident that I knew what to do and what to look for to best care for her when we went home and after the monitor came off.

There is no manual, no wealth of data to tell us what we could expect for one born so young. We have faced many challenges, experienced many triumphs, and are surprised every day with her progress, her gifts and talents. At the time of this writing, Kayla is 19 years old and although she is living a relatively normal life, *there are still challenges and we work every day at finding the best way we can support her life needs in preparation for her to make a successful transition to independence. Kayla was the youngest baby to survive in the state of Oregon in 1999. Advances in medical technologies have improved survival statistics for preemies, even for babies born as early as 23 weeks.*

My goal in sharing this information with you is to provide some insights and information about an NICU experience that will empower you as a parent, family member or friend to be able to better navigate this experience. You are in good hands.

You Are Where You Need to Be

If you have found yourself in a Neonatal Intensive Care Unit, otherwise known as the NICU (or some say nick-you), you are most likely experiencing a full range of emotions and are struggling with how to manage them. Rarely do people anticipate that they will find themselves here, but now that you're here, know that you are in the best place possible. You are in the hands of the Top Guns, the Dream Team of doctors, nurses, respiratory therapists, and caregivers. They are trained and experienced in this type of work. Know that they are dedicated to not only provide the best care to your child, but they are there to prepare you to care for your child as well.

Whether you are expecting to spend a day, a week, or a number of months in the NICU, it is a stressful, unfamiliar, and uncomfortable experience. Trust that you will find your stride. You'll learn what the bells and signals mean and don't mean, and you'll learn a lot about the nature of your child. What's important is to take the urge to focus on fear, and channel it into observation and inquiry. If you don't understand what's happening with your child's care, ask. Educate yourself. The knowledge will reduce your fear and enable you to better partner with your child's caregivers.

The greatest piece of advice I offer you is to observe and be present with your child. Get to know their behaviors, listen for the differences in their cries. Identify changes in their behavior. It can make a crucial difference in their care. The caregivers have several children to care for, but you have only yours. Your knowledge and observations about your child can provide important insights to the care team in how they approach their care strategies.

You will experience ups and downs, good days and not so good days during your stay in the NICU. Your wellbeing is very important to your ability to handle these fluctuations. Remember to breathe. Remember to eat! Remember to take some time for yourselves.

You may feel alone on this journey, but your family and friends are experiencing it too. They may be trying to figure out what they could do to help and have no ideas. The load you are carrying may seem very heavy.

Allow them to lighten it in some way. It may be as simple as picking up your mail, grabbing something for you at the store, bringing you some lunch or meeting you for lunch. If you are comfortable with this, you may even want to allow someone to be your "communications director" to keep everyone updated.

The important thing to remember is that your child is in the best place they can be to receive the care they need. You're in good hands.

EDUCATE YOURSELF

Knowledge reduces fear. Notice, I didn't say "gets rid of". When you think about it, we fear things we have never experienced or don't know much about. Take driving, for instance. When we're growing up, we see our parents driving and blindly trust that they know what they're doing. When we first considered the thought of driving, we encountered fear because we didn't know enough to be comfortable with it. Just like knowing the rules of the road reduces the fear of driving, the experience of driving also tends to lessen the fear. We learn how to spot trouble and avoid dangerous situations. Now, I know this is not the same, but there are some parallels we can draw from this example.

For us, the best way we found to deal with difficult situations was to find out as much as we could about the risks, what was at stake and what to look for that might indicate a concern or problem. Ask questions! The more you know, the better off you are at knowing how to recognize and/or deal with the potential problem. Potential is the key word.

Most situations in the NICU involve the use of technical equipment, tubes, and sensors. For non-technical people, it can be intimidating. Yes, the equipment is very sophisticated, but the displays and sounds are designed to communicate information quickly so that staff can assess and respond quickly and appropriately.

Ask them to tell you what they look for and how the different numbers and levels relate to each other. It may take some time to understand, but you'll get a feel for it. The staff may look at the monitors first, but the real story is generally confirmed by what the child looks like – ask them what you should be looking for – like a change in skin color, lip color, nail beds, do they look uncomfortable, are they showing any behavior that is unusual.

The doctors try to prepare us for the worst-case scenario. It's for our own good. The best-case scenario is what everyone is working toward and being able to take the child home. You don't get to take the doctors and nurses home with you, but you can reduce the fear of caring for the child at home with the knowledge you receive in the NICU.

STATISTICS ARE NUMBERS WITHOUT A SOUL

It is the doctor's responsibility to advise you of the known risks and possible outcomes related to your child's condition. This is based on what is known of the general population and past outcomes. If you've seen pharmaceutical advertisements on the TV, it's much the same. It is supposed to educate you, but often times, it scares you to death! This is their responsibility, but they know that there are many factors at play and each individual person is going to have differences in their responses to treatment.

Mark Twain said, "There are lies, damn lies, and then there are statistics." Statistics are numbers – pieces of data. They have no personality. They don't take into consideration the nature of the individual, how much prayer plays into the situation, the prenatal care received, family support, pure random luck, or the determination of the child's spirit! According to statistics, our daughter shouldn't be here, but she is here and she is thriving. The statistics are meant to give you a big picture view, but they can't predict what will happen with your child.

Statistics don't mean to be unkind or discouraging, or even encouraging. They are numbers without a soul and the soul is a powerful force.

CELEBRATING LIFE VERSUS WARDING OFF DEATH

Just as the effect of a smile is uplifting and a frown brings you down, the positive attitude (and negative attitude) can be felt by those around you – your baby, the nurses, doctors, other parents and their children. Every parent who has a baby in the NICU, be it for a few days, weeks, or months is experiencing a life and death feeling. It is a very deep, emotional experience. When the energy you concentrate on is the celebration of life, it makes the ups and downs a little easier to take.

It is important to internalize that the current moment is all we are guaranteed. Living in the moment is something that is difficult to do in our fast-paced world. Taking the time to really experience the child, or any person in our lives, will reveal many treasures you never knew were there! It is how we should live each day. Savor the moments you have, not the ones you anticipate having or not having.

Every baby has a purpose and a profound impact on both our lives and on those who are close to us. Even in the case of one's death, their purpose can be the

lessons they teach to us about how precious and

unpredictable life can be. Their spirits are precious and

should be celebrated with every moment. In doing so,

we reduce our sense of regret for not having savored

the time we have to spend with them.

COMMUNICATING WITH FRIENDS AND FAMILY

Communicating status updates can be stressful for both you and your friends and family. They are not able to stay current with the everyday events. They are waiting for the phone to ring but may be afraid of what they might hear when the call comes. When the phone rings and they see that the call is from you, address the status directly by starting the conversation with, "he/she's fine", or "he/she's okay", assuring them that the fight is still on. Once they know this, they will be more relaxed and open to receiving whatever details you have to report.

This strategy can be very helpful in any accident or status report that involves people's lives, such as in the event of a car accident or a family member being in the hospital. We have incorporated this method throughout our family and it has made a significant difference to all of us. To state it rather bluntly, once they know that the person is still alive, they will be more capable of actually hearing the report that you are about to give. Starting with anything else leaves the listening on pins and needles to know the answer to their ultimate question as to whether they are alive or not.

IT'S NOT ABOUT ME!

Any parent in this situation struggles with their own emotional stability. Many question their ability to handle the situation, but trust that you will discover strength you never knew you had! The title of this section may be a bit misleading, but the perspective is what is important. It's about what you have to give. As stewards for our children, that is our role, to give them what they need and our support is one of the most critical things we can give.

For a mother, she has a special role to fulfill that few others can. Mother's milk is a very powerful gift. You may not be able to breastfeed a newborn and pumping for breastmilk can be frustrating, time consuming, and can be painful, but every drop is like liquid gold, especially for a challenged baby. There are nutrients in the milk that the child cannot get in any other way. What's a few months in light of a child's lifetime? The comfort in knowing that we are serving a good purpose can go a long way in relieving the feelings of helplessness that can come over you. As it did for me, providing breastmilk can bring much satisfaction as a mother to know you are doing something for your baby that no one else can, and when your baby's as small as mine was, it was one of the only things I could do for her besides just loving her.

In some cases, no matter how hard they try, some mothers are unable to produce breast milk or are unable to sustain the supply needed. There are options available. There are breast milk banks that provide milk for babies, not only in the NICU, but for all babies. Check with your care staff to find out more about the availability of breast milk for your baby, if needed.

So, what about fathers and siblings? Letting the baby hear your voice, touching them, holding them is a support that you can give and even though it is hard to measure, it is known to be beneficial to the wellbeing of the baby. Skin to skin time, referred to as kangaroo care, has proven to be very effective for both the baby and the parent. The warmth of the body, smell of the skin, and sound of the heart beat are all comforting for the child and the parent. I can't tell you how many times my baby fell asleep on her daddy during kangaroo care. Dad got some sleep too! Looking at *the monitor with all its lights and numbers and lines, I could see that there was an evenness to the measurements, the baby was calm. That feeling transferred to me as well.*

There are restrictions for siblings in the NICU for the protection of all the children in the unit but check with your care staff to see what can be done or under what conditions the siblings can have time and interaction with the baby. The siblings may have a hard time believing they have a new brother or sister. Letting them know they have an important role to play as a brother or sister will make the situation more real and can inspire them to participate in some way. Even if they are not able to visit the baby, allowing them to contribute will make a big difference. They could do a phone recording of themselves, singing a song or just talking to the baby. Saying a prayer for them, drawing a special picture to hang near the crib, or allowing them to come up with their own creative way to contribute will help them to feel a part of the baby's life and the family's efforts to support the baby.

If the focus is on what we can give as support to the baby or to those caring for the child, the tendency to focus on how hard this is for us becomes less. Knowing we are making a difference for the child's welfare is priceless.

WRITE IT DOWN

Keeping a daily journal can prove to be helpful and therapeutic. There are so many emotions and activities that happen every day and after a time, it may become hard to recall specific events, procedures, or therapies that were performed that you may be asked about at a later time. Yes, the medical records should reflect these events, but they are not always easily accessible when the need arises.

Journaling can be a great outlet for expression. It's not a matter of writing pages of thoughts, but it's a journey and just like any other journey you take, after a time, we forget so much about the journey, but when we journal about it, we can revisit what it was like at that moment and we discover just how much of the journey we have forgotten.

I journaled every day during my time in the NICU. That was 142 days. In it, I expressed my state of mind, my struggles, my fears, my moments of joy, my triumphs. I know I just said it was not about me, but this was my way of finding and honoring myself and my struggle, my journey, as it related to my baby's journey. It was a way for me to unload my burden without impacting anyone around me and I could spend as much or as little time as I needed to get those feelings out.

Good, bad, or indifferent, these are the moments we're living. Even recalling the hardships that we may face can show us how far we've come and see how the tough times can make us stronger and wiser. That goes for our babies too! No matter how long the journey in the NICU, time seems to move at a snail's pace. When we look back, we can see their accomplishments and celebrate their overcoming struggles and fighting for life.

If we can then use that new found strength to help others going through the same thing, the price we pay for that hardship or struggle becomes less. We can also see the beauty of small victories and the ways we were able to overcome doubt and fear.

Share Your Story

Being in the NICU, you may feel like you are an island, but when you share your story, you will most likely be surprised at how many people have an NICU story of their own or of someone they know. Knowing someone else is or has gone through a similar situation is comforting. If you're new to the NICU, talk to those who have been there for a while. If you've been there for a while, recognize when new parents arrive and take a moment to introduce yourself, letting them know they are not alone.

We may read stories in the paper or hear them on TV, but it is different when something like this happens to someone you know. Sharing your story with friends and family can have a profound impact. Not only are they interested in your wellbeing and that of your child, but they also tend to take a moment and reflect on their own lives and that of their own children. They may also have stories to share that can help you.

In sharing our story with friends who had a baby a few months after ours, we helped them to be able to deal with the news of their baby having a terminal genetic disease. They educated themselves to prepare for what lay ahead and they were able to celebrate every moment of his short, precious life. This goes back to the idea that this experience is not just for us as parents. It extends much farther than we could ever imagine, touching many lives and many hearts along the way.

I'm not suggesting that we should broadcast everything about the experience to everyone, but holding it inside can deprive you or someone else from bits of knowledge or wisdom that could be vital to someone who is or will be going through a similar situation.

WORK WITH YOUR SUPPORT TEAM

Know that if you are here and your baby came early or is needing extra help to overcome some challenge, there's no better place that you or your baby could be.

The staff...all of the staff are dedicated, talented, compassionate, loving people who care about you as a parent and for your successful journey home. They love each and every one of these babies as if they were their own.

Procedures and events that occur in the NICU require quick and focused response. As parents, our instinct is to jump in and help. Cool heads and expertise are what is called for in these situations. Our job as parents is to try to control our emotions, stand back, and allow the professionals to do what they do best. Having said that, this would be the time to share any behaviors that you may have observed that are out of the ordinary. This input can be helpful to the staff in making an accurate assessment of the situation. But, if asked to clear the room, it is important to respect their wishes so they can do what is required.

During your stay, you will work with many different caregivers with differing styles and personalities. Although their training and knowledge may be the same, their interpersonal skills and manner of delivering care may differ. For instance, two teachers may deliver the same curriculum, but their style of delivery may be different. You may prefer the style of one over the other, yet your best friend has the opposite preference. These differences are inevitable in any population of people. Learn what works best for you and let your staff know. It may not always be possible to accommodate your preference, but if known, your preferences can be considered when staff assignments are made.

The babies develop so quickly and their needs and behaviors change over time. Methods that worked previously may no longer be working and other methods may need to be used. Even trying something that didn't work before may prove to be successful now. Being flexible is important. In the area of basic care, there is no definitive right or wrong way for each child. One may not consider creativity to be something of value in medical care, but creativity can reveal new *and effective methods in the area of basic care such as feeding, bathing, holding, and comforting. Being open to trying new or different methods can prove to be very beneficial. You may even have ideas of your own that you would like to try. Discuss it with your caregiver.*

Trust in your team. Learn from them, thank them. Establish a relationship with your caregivers. Communication is very important for calming fear through knowing more about who you are working with and how you can better work together for the overall success of your child's treatment. They work hard under difficult conditions and yet they put themselves on the line every day for our children. It is a calling that brings them to this type of work. They are your constant ally.

Some families don't have an NICU near their home and have to travel many miles to be able to spend time with their baby at the NICU. There may be a home available, suited for you and families like yours so that you can visit and stay whenever possible. Help is available and comes in many forms, so don't hesitate to ask. If you need help with lactation (breastfeeding), would like to plug into a support group, need spiritual guidance or support, or to know of available literature or other resources, talk to your care staff for the services available within the facility as well as those that are available in the area where you live. When you establish care with your pediatrician, be sure to ask about the additional services that may be available once you have taken your child home.

Your support team will help you in whatever way they can. You may not be able to take in all the information the first time it is given, but ask them to repeat it for you. They understand that it is a lot to take in. They are going to do what they can to ensure that you are as confident as possible when you take your baby home. Although it doesn't happen as much as they would like, take a moment from time to time to let them know how you are doing. They love to hear from you.

FROM OUR FAMILY WITH LOVE...

Believe in yourself.

Believe you have the strength to meet this challenge.

Believe that you were chosen for this experience.

Believe in the Creator's grace,

And search for the lessons you are to carry with you and share with others.

Thank you for allowing us to share our experience and some of the lessons we have learned. Our warmest prayers and thoughts go out to all NICU babies, parents, families, and staff.